I0413848

STIFF

JULES蘇

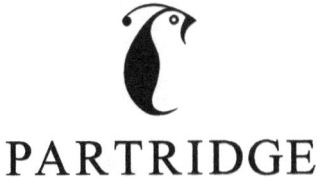

PARTRIDGE

Copyright @ 2022 by Jules蘇.

Project Marshal by PiPi的姐姐
Construction by Liz & CW
Doodles by Kok Bee

ISBN: Softcover   978-1-5437-6454-3
             eBook   978-1-5437-6455-0

All rights reserved. No part of this book may be used or reproduced by
any means, graphic, electronic or mechanical, including photocopying,
recording, taping or by any information storage retrival system without
the written permission of the author expect in the case of brief quotations
embodied in critical articles and reviews.

Because of the dynamic nature of the Internet, any web addresses or links
contained in this book may have changed since publication and may no
longer be valid. The views expressed in this work are solely those of the
author and do not necessarily reflect the views of the publisher, and the
publisher hereby disclaims any responsibility for them.

Print information available on the last page.

To order additional copies of this book, contact
Toll Free +65 3165 7531 (Singapore)
Toll Free +60 3 3099 4412 (Malaysia)
orders.singapore@partridgepublishing.com

www.partridgepublishing.com/singapore

REPETITIONS

Sweat - 1ml

You would be asking what is "Sweat 0 ml?" This is how the chapters will be defined by the ml (millilitres) of sweat for each chapter as "Little Student" goes along her journey. Who is "Little Student"? Is she a ten year old??? Haha No… definitely not. Let me introduce you to "Little Student".

Main Character : Little Student

Age : Mid 40s almost late 40s (let's not be so specific about this as this is obviously not an important factor)

Gender : Passionate, driven lioness aka… female

Lifestyle : Busy working schedule, late nights, starts her day early and fingers contentedly on a "treadmill", achievable km per day – maybe 3km or more (something to figure out later)

Nickname : Lil' Student

This experience is about Lil' Student finding a new passion and going through a life-changing period. She wants to share this with anyone and hopes that it will also bring these changes to their lives too. What she is trying to achieve is to share an experience out there to all that would like to take good care of themselves and always think that 'fitness' is such a big deal with all the shiny machines, weights that can break a toe if you drop it, all the intimidating classes where people are shouting and just moving so fast (jumping, skipping or even dancing are done at such high speed and intensity). All the humans in this place are "huge" or of a certain size with bulging extra flesh which are called "muscles". All that is what you will find in a place called "The Gym" and yes this is where we will start Lil' Student's journey of 12 months (when this was written).

Lil' Student wanted to start to feel strong and not be catching her breath after a flight of stairs (yes this seems to be the definition that everyone uses right but it is so so true). So what's next? And how to do this? Lil' Student does not like sports at all and has not done any sports at all and just basically does not like to sweat. So Lil' Student went to the GYM one day and was determined to do all the things that people do in a GYM. So Lil' Student signed up and errr… where does she start??? So she decided to sign up for a Personal Training program to start off and thinking that ok she will just learn a lot from the 10 lessons signed up but ohh… boy…. How wrong she was, haha. From 10 lessons now it's been almost 24 months and many many 10 lessons have gone by and Lil' Student is still learning.

And as much as Lil' Student predicted her Trainer is 6ft tall and she is literally invisible in height and width. He is one of the Huge Guys that we see on brochures and TV. But Lil' Student remained calm and told herself "it's ok, he is just tall and she will get used to him soon".

Soon it was Lil' Student's first session/training and it was more of an assessment session to see where Lil' Student stands. Of course everything was "new" and everything felt exciting because it's new and there was no "level" that was needed to be fulfilled. And plus of course Mr. Trainer was super nice (first time of course he was, wait for the real "Mr. Trainer" – later in Sweat Chapters). It was February 2019 when it all began.

Sweat - 2ml

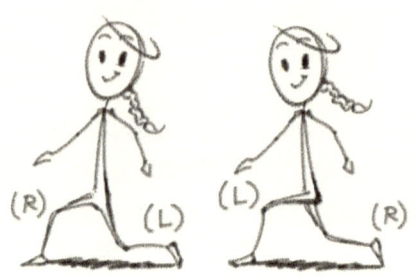

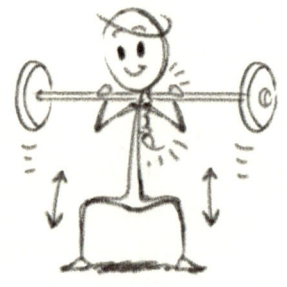

So Lil' Student started her first session and this is what happened.

Mr. Trainer – Ok now we will do the Squat (the one and only ever famous Squat, it's a must do or a must have like a "that shade of Lipstick").

Lil' Student – Ok looking very confident and just stood there and paid 100% attention to Mr. Trainer's demo and ok looks easy enough. But after my first squat – all I'm hearing was this:

- Ok, push your glutes (what is even "Glutes" OMG – it's your butt) behind when you go down. What??? Push my butt behind??? How do you do that? Ok never mind I will try and almost sat on my butt on the floor. Ok after a few tries better and nowhere there at all, and then now I have to worry about Knees cannot exceed your Feet.... This is just too much to brain when you are trying to push your butt behind and at the same time need to make sure your Knees do not exceed your Feet.... Can we just do 1 thing at a time??? I guess not, both have to be done together.

So I learned a way to register all these moves, names etc by converting it into my own understandable terms.

Squat – "think like a Duck or more like you are the Duck and stick your butt out and squat and eventually you will get it". Once you do this right, your knees will automatically not exceed your feet.

Squat – perfected this to 80% verified by Mr. Trainer, after 5 sessions and that would be around 1 month as we do not do squats for every session.

Definition:

Lil' Student – Butt/bottom
Muscle World – Glutes

Mr. Trainer – next is the Squat's best buddy which is the "Lunges" for some reason these 2 come hand in hand and are the first basic things you will learn but it will stay with you forever as till today I have to do Squats and Lunges – basically you will never graduate from it but will be with weights and longer distances for Lunges – like you can do Lunges from the GYM to the next door Shop and back – buy an Ice-Cream maybe??

Lunges is a movement where you place 1 leg in front and bend the knee to 90° and repeat on the other side.

Lil' Student – Omg my thighs hurt!! How to do it 10 times each side? I won't be able to walk out of the gym later. And the next line will be – OMG I can't get up – please help me!!! How do you do this??? But all I'm getting is just a Voice counting – 1, 2...... 3...... 4...... and no one is hearing my OMG(s)....

Lunges – this is no conversion figured till today – it is still Lunges....

Lunges – finally can manage 10 times each side in April – 80% fewer comments from Mr. Trainer means it's good to go ya....

Definition:

Lil' Student – Thighs/Drumsticks
Muscle World – Quads

Mr. Trainer – Burpees – what are burpees?? It's another dying move. Breathe, breathe, put your hands behind your head and take deep breaths.... Lil' Student... speechless as she is trying to catch her breath....

Burpees – an explosive move that is a total body workout. You start with a Plank, legs jump forward towards your body and stand up and jump up with hands in the air and then back on "four" and Legs jump back to a Plank position again and continue. This move is normally done only 10 times and that also will leave you breathless.... And this move also does not leave you, it will come back every now and then but maybe more in counts/reps.

Definition

Lil' Student – Counts/how many times
Muscle World – reps means repetitions

Mr. Trainer – **Step Board Jump** – we are not done yet –
1 more last exercise. You just need to jump on the Step
Board with 2 feet together.

Lil' Student – ok finally something easy – just jump only
and the Step Board is super low, how hard could it be
compared to all the above right? I was so so wrong. I could
not jump with BOTH feet on the Step Board. Yes I couldn't
even believe it myself – how is that possible right? Just
jump only on the Stepper but I keep landing with 1 Feet
after the other.

Managed to finally jump with BOTH feet landed at the
same time after 2 sessions!!! And the Step Board will never
look the same ever. It is not just a Step Board – it's evil
hahaha....

Sweat - 3ml

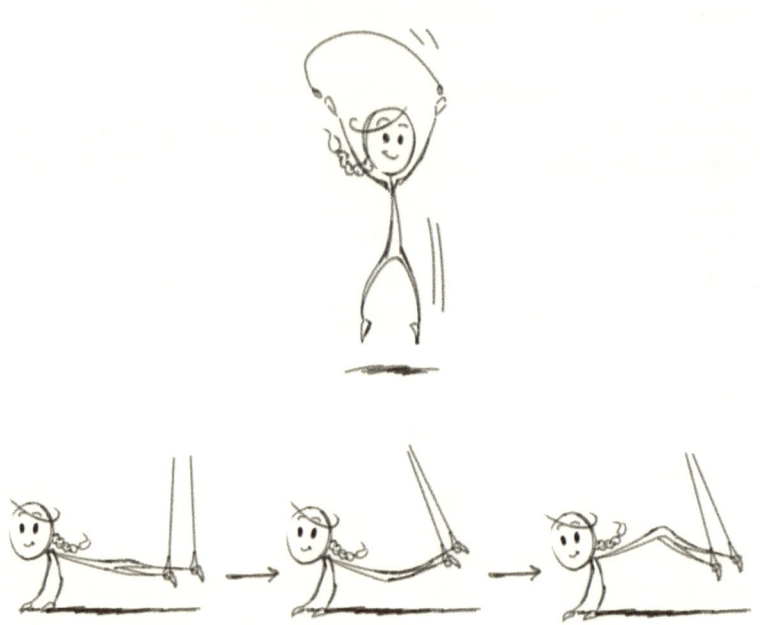

Now next Sweat Session

Mr. Trainer – so we have met Ms. Squat, Mr. Lunges, Tough Burpees and Evil Step Board. What do we have next? (with a big Smile as usual, so deceiving). Let's do something normal and simple… (this is when I will turn around and roll my eyes… like as if I will believe you right?).

Jump Rope – simple enough and it's familiar ground, all of us have done this since school days, but I was so wrong again and yes everyone please keep count of how many times I will be repeating this, literally to the end of this book.

This is the Real Jump Rope, the Jump Rope that Adults do or does everyone? Or maybe I'm the only one that cannot do this...You are supposed to jump BOTH Legs again... and I think BOTH Legs is the problem (same as Evil Step Board). I COULD NOT do this, I COULD not jump with BOTH Legs and I kept Jump Rope with alternate Legs. It's ok to keep trying but after 5 times, both Mr. Trainer and I said "ok let's put this aside and we will come to this sometime later ya".

Lil' Student – not that proud of this achievement but it is still an achievement and it deserves to be documented – ok finally did this after 4 tries in between and did it in October (you do the math – reminder this journey started in February).

Mr. Trainer – now let's go to **The World of Steel – Deadlift (12.5kgs)**. Ok now do not get excited this is not the Barbell that you see on TV and lifting it above your head (not there yet...) this is a Steel Bar and lifted from the ground with Knees slightly bent (The Duck Move needs to happen here again) + Chest Out (like a Pigeon) + Shoulder rotate backward – yes all must be done at the same time and lift up straight and down to the Shin.

Pike – this is a Friend from TRX... which is a class that I attend. These are workouts with Straps and depending on the workout – it could be your legs or your hands in the Straps. TRX is not part of the Sweat Sessions but I work with Mr. Trainer to perfect this move. You start with your legs in the Strap and in Plank position – and you push your body upwards till your body is like upside down "U" and you straighten your body.

Lil' Student – Did it after 2 months!!

Mr. Trainer – now we go to the rounder side of Things – **The Medicine Ball – Slam Ball** is the correct name and I found out much later. This is a Ball filled with Sand and it has different weights. What do you do with it? Super simple, just lift it up above your head and throw it down with all your might… (I know what you are thinking and yes you are right… think of someone that you do not like and I bet you can really throw it down hard…). So if you are curious when I do this – I think of Mr. Trainer and most of the time this is one of the well done exercises!!! One of the most satisfying exercises especially after you are 30 mins into your Sweat Session – yes you do feel like throwing something at someone but in this case, slam it to the ground!!

Mr. Trainer – now let's meet **"Battling Rope"** yes it did not get its name for no reason. You will need to hold the Thick Rope and make waves. You are supposed to be creating a Tidal Wave like a Mini Tsunami but Lil' Student's version was just small waves like by the shore on a day without any wind…. But I will get there one day to create the Tidal Wave.

Notes:

Weight Gain
After weeks of workout, you will find that you will put on some weight which is so confusing right when you spend hours and hours sweating in the GYM and here your weight goes up!! Do not panic! Remain calm. There is a reason behind it.

Exercise = Muscle Soreness = Micro Tears = Healing = Water Retention for Healing

You should not look at the Total Weight but pay more attention to Muscle Mass gain.

Always switch to a different routine throughout the week as the same routine would mean you are only working out the same muscles.

Day 1 – Upper Body
Day 2 – Leg Day
Day 3 – Cardio, HIIT

My Routine for the first 12 months:

- 2 days of Training – combination of the above
- 2 days of TRX (Strength and Core) whenever possible
- 1 day of Zumba (for coordination which is so so bad that I even laugh at myself silly in class)

Isolation means – only 1 part of the muscle is being worked out on 1 type of exercise.

Compound means – few muscles are being worked out with just 1-2 types of exercise.

Progressive Overload (sensitive word) – need to do this whenever possible to increase intensity and push your body further as your body will not progress if you keep doing it with the same intensity.

Soreness – meet your constant companion that will stay with you side by side for months, like it or not. Sometimes it's kind but at times, you do not even own your Body anymore. Walking down the stairs after Leg Day was such a pain and it felt like I was 90 years old and yes even my neighbor aunty was faster than me so I had to pretend that

I injured my Leg....

But wait, when this happens there is a solution to lessen the pain...

- Hot Press – make your own. Old socks filled with beans and micro for 1 min and press on sore for not more than 5 mins and max 4 times a day (approved by Mr. Trainer).
- This stage will not last forever and as you progress Soreness will lessen and you will start to miss it yes, you will miss it.

Sweat - 4ml

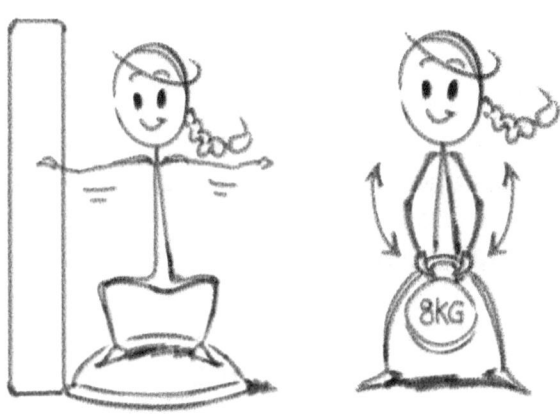

Sweat Session – Bosu, Kettlebell, Push-up, Sit-up, Sandbag

Mr. Trainer – We have done Jump Rope, Pike, Slam Ball and Battle Rope, let's move on….

Bosu Squat – this is like a half moon Ball filled with air, you will need to balance on it and actually this has become one of my Fav, it's quite fun though the first time, I did more of a "Wobbling Dance" vs a "Squat on the Bosu". This is very good for balancing.

Stand against a pillar (beginner) and balance yourself on Bosu and start squatting + doing the wobbling dance…

Nothing was achieved… must say it was quite ok simply because 1 hand was on the pillar. But of course right… no way I could have balance and squat on this wobbling platform….

Kettlebell Swing – yes this literally looks like a Kettle, a very heavy kettle but without the spout.

Hold the handle with both hands, stand with feet apart and move your Hips back and front as you swing the Kettlebell in between your Legs. Status now – still cannot swing with just Hips but swinging more using Arms and Body which is totally wrong, wrong. I cannot brain 2 actions at the same time if you notice – back to coordination – will take me some time to do this right. One point to know if you are not doing it right will be – your lower back will hurt.

Achieved and did it right after a month… and just swing your Hips and squeeze your Glutes aka… Butt.

Series of Burpees, Push-up and Sit-up – ok managed this and still smiling.

Sandbag Slam – we do this exercise that is called "Fireman" and this Sandbag looks like a Bolster and we carry it on the shoulder and drop it to the back, turn around and lift up to shoulder and drop it again and continue… the weight was manageable as it was not that heavy but try turning round and round and after 5 times… my world was spinning!

Snacks – month of May. There were no snacks on my Desk – no chips at all and what I see are "Quaker Squares" and Granola(s)… what happened??? This will happen once you start this journey.

When you walk around the supermarket and you stand in front of a shelf of chips but you just stare and you do not buy any when you check out – you are on the right path. Self control… even till today I still do this, I would stand in front of all the Chips and just see what flavours there are but walk out without purchasing any and so proud of myself.

Shorts – downgrade from "M" to "S" but be mindful that your weight may still be the same but your physique will be more toned. Getting tone does not necessarily mean "losing weight" at least not for me.

Sweat - 5ml

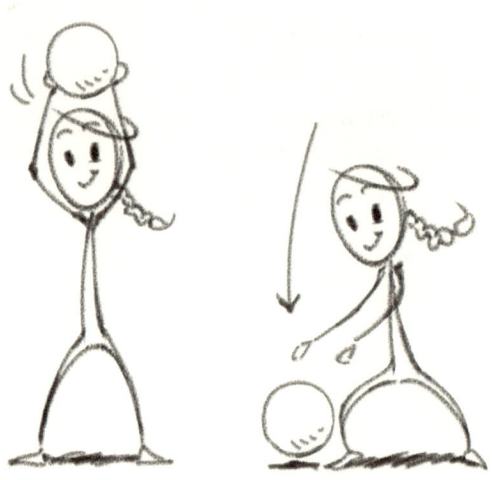

Sweat Session – Slam Ball, Cycling (Assault Bike), Step Board Jump

Mr. Trainer – It's May now it's time to try more fusion moves (means basic with diversions…).

Skater with Medicine Ball (Dancing Move) – please do not be mistaken, this is totally not a dancing move. Hold the Ball at your chest level and jump side to side with 1 Leg under the other like a Curtsy position. Reps were 12 times x 2 sets.

Lil' Student – already struggling with a "Huge Ball" in my hand and alternating Legs but 'I HAD TO DO IT WITH STYLE!!!??" After a while not sure which Leg is supposed to be where and was it right or left – HELP!!!! When you do it slowly you can coordinate Legs and Hands and balance the Ball but when slow – there is NO STYLE… now I know why it's called the Dancing Move in a way.

Mr. Trainer – ok that's it you got it right, now do it with STYLE and the minute he says that – all goes wrong… never mind we will try and get better next time ok….

Dancing Move – nothing was achieved… totally NO STYLE was achieved!

Assault Bike – this is a Bicycle that has a Huge Wheel in front and it has a fan that actually blows air as you cycle. Another very deceiving machine as in order, to get the Air blowing, you are the ONE that is doing the work. If you want the Air to blow faster, then you will need to cycle faster… which explains the name – Assault Bike – it does assault you in a way… till you are out of breath. But this is considered a fair machine as you work harder and you get rewarded with cool Air. And this exercise is normally by seconds. Now I need to emphasize seconds here, seconds to us are just a flick of a finger and it's a few seconds gone but not when you are exercising: the seconds feel like minutes… 10s sounds short but again it is not, trust me when you are exercising and out of breath – it feels forever…

– nothing much to achieve as this is just cycling pretty easy but I need to improve on the speed, cycle faster.

Dancing Move 2 (Skater to Half Burpees Ball Slam) – another Ball Dancing Move – hold the Ball and jump to the side, slam the Ball down and drop your body to the floor to Burpee's similar move (jump back and forth while hands on Ball).

Step Board Jump – yes the Stepper is back – this time stand with open legs on both side of the Step Board and jump on it (please land softly and not like a "Hippo") but that's what I did, landed so hard with full might hahaha... and then jump back to original position, did this 5 times. Next time Plank on Step Board **(elbow on the floor and legs placed on the step board)** and do Mountain Climb x 5 times x 2 sets.

Mountain Climb – this is done with Full Plank and you tuck your knees in and out – alternate legs at a time – kind of like "speed running" on Full Plank.

At this point my sweat is already dripping. Nicely done!

You must be wondering about Mr. Trainer by now, and yes Mr. Trainer is super big vertically and horizontally, means he is very Tall, very muscular and very intimidating but he is such a "Gentle Giant" and with his patience and guidance and enough breath to keep repeating every move like at least 3 times (as I cannot remember by the time he does more than 1 move hahaha...). It's been 2 months now and still going strong. And as time goes by I slowly learned to trust Mr. Trainer and start to see the benefit of this and plus all the silly mistakes that I do, we always end up doing extra ABS exercises (laughing). By now I'm beginning to enjoy my training, starting to learn and trying very hard to remember what I learn.

At this point I'm still struggling to try to eat healthier and trying to make Oats my next best friend to have, especially at night when I get hungry and for mornings. Started to make my own Overnight Oats with the help from another Trainer and I know we all do not really like Oats right but it is actually not that bad and I'm starting to like it as it's so easy and convenient for someone like me who really does not have time to prepare breakfast. Now I just do this and grab a jar and off to work and I never miss breakfast.

Sweat - 6ml

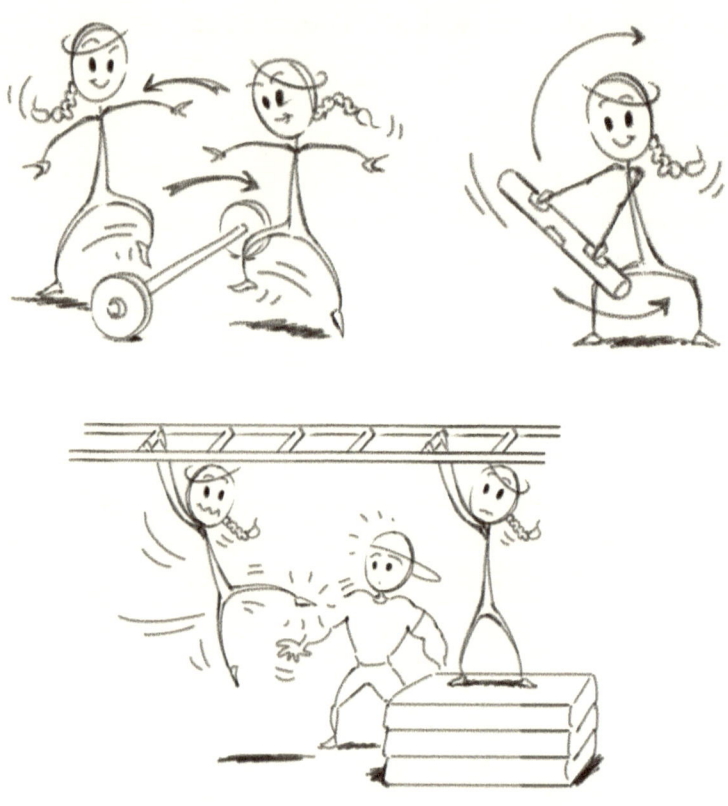

Sweat Session – Circuit, Kettlebell, aka... Charlie Chaplin Move, ViPR, Sandbag, Monkey Bar

Mr. Trainer – Today we will try some new moves and Circuit

1. **Side to Side Burpees** – place a barbell in the center and start to do side by side (jumping) burpees with the barbell as the barrier.
2. **ViPR (8kg)** – this is like a Pipe or tube with holes on

each side and this is where you hold the ViPR. You lift with both hands from the ground to above your head – up and down x 10 times. Sounds easy again but after 10 times x 3 sets, it's no longer easy.

3. **Sandbag (10kg)** – run from Point 1 to Point 2, lift Sandbag and carry on right shoulder and run to Point 1, drop Sandbag and lift to left shoulder and run to Point 2 and keep repeating and this is done by seconds. Wow you are strong now, this 10kgs = 1 bag of Rice.

4. **Kettlebell Swing** – and yes did it nicely and correctly x 10 times x 3 sets. Well done!

5. **Single Dumbbell Windmill** – aka Charlie Chaplin Move (tempo) - this move must be done with Mr. Trainer humming the Charlie Chaplin song. Hold the dumbbell straight up with your right hand and bend your body to the side (left) and straighten back up, do 10 times each side x 3 sets.

Monkey Bar

We all know what a Monkey Bar is – we had this in the playground when we were growing up but a Monkey Bar in the Gym is much higher, I cannot reach it even on tip toe. I have to use the Stepper plus tip toe, in order to reach it.

How it is supposed to be done? You are supposed to be hanging on the Bar and only your hand moves from Bar to Bar while your Legs are supposed to be just hanging down.

Reality, this is what happened: while I was hanging on the Bar, I couldn't control my Legs and they are swaying all over the place while I'm trying to hang on to the Bar and trying to make the 1 Move to the next Bar and end up kicking Mr. Trainer in the event and only managed to move just 1 Bar.

<u>Cautious Note</u> to all Trainers out there. If you ever have a new student doing this, please wear a Sumo Suit to protect yourself as you will be kicked.

Mr. Trainer – at this point I think he is super stressed as he was trying very hard to avoid being kicked but at the same time he cannot be too far away from me, as he needs to make sure I'm safe and do not fall off from the Bar.

Ok we are done for today and it has been quite a while since we did this again haha. I think I will not be allowed to do this till I'm stronger and able to control my Legs better. Well I'm sorry, first time trying ok, I will get better one day.

Sweat - 7ml

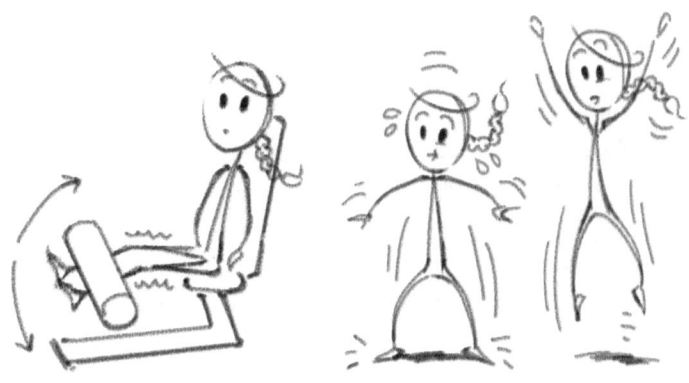

Sweat Session Treadmill, Leg Extension Machine, Dumbbell Squat, Jump Squats, Jumping Jacks, Smith Machine (push), Abs – Sit-up(s)

Mr. Trainer – Let's Go!

1. **Treadmill** – this is the "warm-up" that we do before every sweat session - normally about 10 mins
2. **Leg Extension (machine)** – you hook your legs to the cushioned bar and lift upwards while sitting down. Did 3 sets but different variance of reps and weights. The heavier the weight the lesser the reps, the lighter the weight the higher the reps. **Set 1 (Heavy) x 10, Set 2 (Medium) x 15, Set 3 (Light) x 18**
3. **Dumbbell Deep Squats (10kg)** – hold dumbbells with both hands and start squatting – Deep Squats means you need to go low, super low x 10 x 3 Sets. I cannot feel my "Drumsticks" by now – sort of disconnected....

4. **Jump Squats** – killer, killer move.... You need to squat and jump and straight back to the squat position and continue for x 10 x 3 sets. This is when you wish your legs had Springs... so you can bounce up and down... with lesser effort.

5. **Jumping Jacks – x 15 x 2 sets** – nicely done but out of breath...

6. **Squats (Smith Machine)** – this is an assisted machine, supposedly when it's assisted it is supposed to be easier right, if not why do you even have that function? No it is not easier, not in any way at all. You hold on to the Bar, middle finger on the line... (yes there is groovy line as guide), go under the Bar so that the Bar rest on your shoulder now, legs forward, lift the Bar off the hook and start squatting x 10 x 3 sets... did quite well I must say and I kind of like this Mr. Smith... and yes it is Mr. Smith till today but of course now... with added weights.... I do not really like it that much anymore, killer move that always kill my Quads (drumsticks).

7. **Sit-up Benches** – as usual we always end our session with ABS. Hook your legs on the Bench and lie down and this bench is declining so your head is at the bottom, legs on top and start to do Sit-ups, normally this should start hurting after 1st set of 10x... and eventually it will be slower and slower but still manage to finish the set... beautifully as always.

Notes:

I'm beginning to realize that the 1 hour seems to go by faster and it feels like 30 mins, is this a sign that I'm enjoying what I do now? By now I'm able to do a proper Squat but will struggle when it's a different exercise and especially with weights, it's a whole different world when weights are added to your workout.

The Different Bells (not the ones that ring ya)....

Dumbbells – not sure till now why they are called dumbbells.
Barbell – to me this is like a longer version of a Dumbbell right?
Ezy Barbell – this one the bar is curvy and looks exactly like a Barbell but with a curvy bar.

Sweat - 8ml

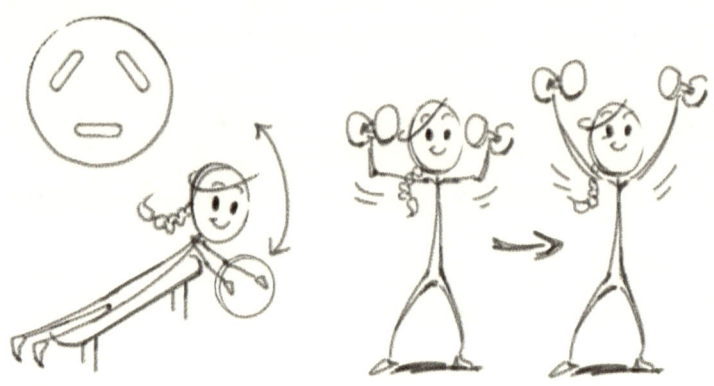

Sweat Session: Shoulder Day

Mr. Trainer – This will be an easy day – a chill day (ya right, he always says this for every session ya).

1. **Dumbbell Military Press – Light (4kgs) x 12 reps x 3 sets** – sit with your lower back firmly against the bench. Keep your shoulders and back as straight as possible. Raise the dumbbells from your thighs and bring them to shoulder height. Push straight up and exhale and bring it down to ear level and inhale. **Heavy (6kgs) x 8 reps x 3 sets.** 1st set was still fine, able to do it on my own, but 2nd and 3rd set you can see the energy is going downhill, and I need Mr. Trainer's assistance, but please don't be mistaken, assistance does not mean he is helping much, just merely with his finger tips only. Thanks…

2. **Shoulder Press Machine** – there are 2 parts to this machine where you place your hands, Outer and

Inner. But of course Inner is always stronger due to the closer gap and Outer range was pretty hard. But still I have to finish my set ya.

3. **Clean and Press – (12kgs)** – lift the Barbell from the ground to shoulder and push upwards above your head and repeat for 10 x 3 sets. Again needed assistance after the 1st set.

4. **Lying Front Raise – (5kgs) x 10 x 3 sets** – you lean on an incline bench and use both hands to hold this plates and it has like 3 holes for you to hold. (hmmm now not sure if it is 2 or 3 holes)… and you lift straight upwards, super hard move and couldn't raise my hand all the way up…

5. **Warrior Plank – Next level of Plank** – alternating between Elbow Plank and Straight Plank…. This is when the water works happen… your sweat will start to drip and yes drip….

6. **Elbow Plank + Mountain Climb** – elbow plank while "sprinting" mount climb.

7. **Abs** – sit-ups + heel touching – you lie down with knees up and come up to touch your heels with your hands.

Notes:

TRX is one of my favourite workouts, challenging but fun and can really make you strong. My signature is my sweat will be in 1 line, yes and this is achievable when you do "push ups" and "back squats". This week was a very productive week as I spent 6 days in the gym until I'm not sure where it aches anymore.

Sweat - 9ml

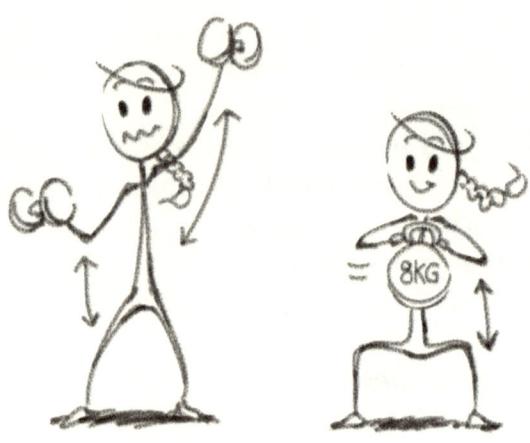

Sweat Session: Battle Rope day +... etc... etc... of course it's never just 1 exercise.

Mr. Trainer – Today we will have so much fun with The Rope! It gets better and better each session... (this is when I start rolling my eyes).

1. **Battling Rope** – remember the Tidal Waves with Wind – yes it's back. I had to do a 20s battle Rope for every move below. But my Tidal Wave has improved. Now it's looking more like a Wave.
2. **Kettlebell Swing – (8kgs) x 10 x 1 set + 20s Battle Rope** – swing your Hips and this move is like Mr. Bean's Dance.
   Mr. Trainer – at the moment you need to make your hips more mobile as your hips are slightly tight. But you will learn and be mobile and soon can join Mr. Bean.

3. **Kettlebell Squat** – **(8kgs) x 10 x 1 set + 20s Battle Rope** – hold the kettlebell and place it near to your chest level and squat. Hands must always be at the center of your body and not at the side or else you will fall backwards. Ok did this well enough and did not fall backwards but anyway even if I do, it's Mr. Trainer is there to ensure that he catches me in time.

4. **Kettlebell Shoulder High Pull** – **(8kgs) x 10 x 1set + 20s Battle Rope** – stand straight and hold the kettlebell with your straight hand down and lift kettlebell all the way up to the chest area with elbows pointed high. Did this very well. Big Smiles all the way… (beyond the smiles the whole time I concentrated more on the kettlebell not hitting my chin…). And suddenly I realized not just the Battle Rope but what's with the 8kgs all the way… Today's workout should be called "Battle Rope 20s and 8kgs Day!!!"

   Mr. Trainer – shoulders getting stronger and deadlift movement is goooddddd…. Impresss (notice there are so many "oooooo"s).

5. **Double Kettlebell Squat** – **(8kgs) x 2 x 10 x 1 set + 20s Battle Rope** – now it's 2 Kettlebells, placed near the chest and squat. I need extra work to hold on to both and do the workout but manage this also with a Smile.

   Mr. Trainer – Well Done!!

6. **Standing Side Crunch with Dumbbell** – **(5kgs) x 6 x 1 set + 20s Battle Rope** – hold and raise dumbbell with 1 hand and bring down so your elbow touches your knees then you raise the hand with dumbbell upwards. Any move that requires lifting and raising my arms is always a problem as my left side has limited motion range… hmmm

could it be that my left side tendons are shorter???? Hahaha… I did not get any answer from Mr. Trainer but just a look….

Mr. Trainer – synchronization needs to improve but balance much better… (means more work needs to be done in a nicer way…).

7. **Single Farmers Walk – (10kgs) + 20s Battle Rope** – this is to stabilize your core when you walk with 1 hand straight at the side – walk in a straight line. Sounds easy but it is not easy. This move you need to do with the Pink Panther Movie song, works best with this move. Do not need any player as Mr. Trainer will hum the tune as I walk.

   Mr. Trainer – left side is weaker than right as right side is dominant if you are right-handed. Don't worry, it can be adjusted later.

Notes:

Today was quite a tough day as you can see besides the normal workout, each move is added with a 20s Battle Rope and this is the killer.

Deep thoughts after this session – if I ever break-in the gym (for whatever reason) The Battle Rope would be the thing that I would make it disappear which means I need to be stronger as I will still need to drag it out of the gym ya… need to give it more thought… maybe a Plan B…

Sweat - 10ml

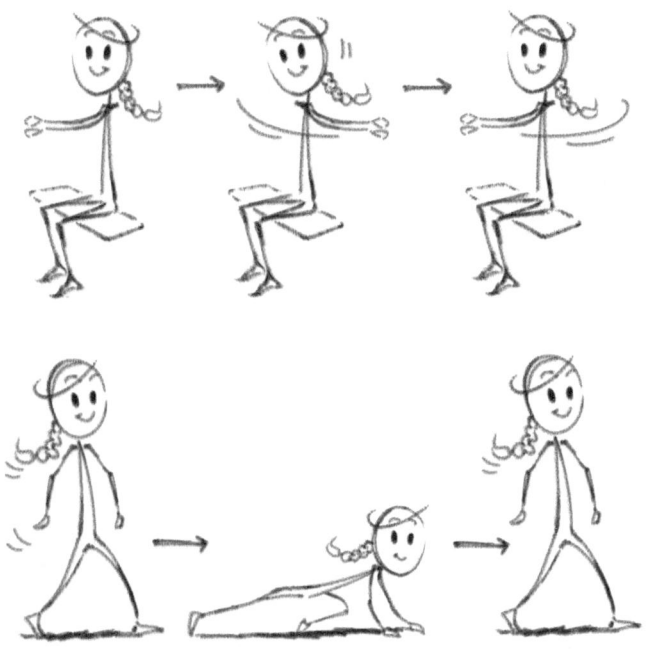

Sweat Session: Circuit – 35s Day

Mr. Trainer – For this we will do this in the TRX room… it's a combination of 4 sets x 4 exercises x 35s each exercise x 3 sets.

Set 1
Mountain Climb (35s)
Plank (35s)
Jump Squat (35s)
Standing Abs Crunch (35s)

Set 2
Burpees (35s)
Side Plank (35s)
Inch Worm (35s)
Push-ups (35s)

Set 3
Wood Chops (35s)
Shoulder Tap Plank (35s)
Frog Squat Tuck (35s)
Russian Twist (35s)

Set 4
V-Tuck (35s)
V-Hold (35s)
Sit Toe Tap (35s)
Warrior Plank (35s)

Rest – 1 min in between

1. **Mountain Climb – 35s** – full Plank position and run on spot.
   Mr. Trainer – core activation is very good.
2. **Elbow Plank – 35s** – this I must say was pretty easy (maybe because it's just the first set).
3. **Jump Squat – 35s** – still a killer till now, must improve on landing with knees bent.
4. **Standing Abs Crunch – 35s** – a coordination move which is right elbow touch left knees, and alternate on both sides. Best done slowly or all energy will be wasted.
5. **Regression Burpees – 35s** – according to Mr. Trainer this is one of my favourite moves. But he was kind today, got a big discount of no need to jump but then still struggled at 5 reps onwards.

6. **Side Plank** – **35s** – this is Plank but on the side and lift 1 arm up and make sure the lifted arm is aligned with the arm below. Tilt the spine bone a bit. Sweat should be starting to drip at this stage.
7. **Inch Worm** – **35s** – this is done by walking with your hands till you are in a Plank position.
8. **Push-ups** – **35s** – still find this very hard and struggle to do this even with knees down.
   Mr. Trainer – still in regression, but technique is good. Slowly but surely she can go for a full push-up without any struggle.
9. **Wood Chops** – **35s** – must be sync! Another coordination move that I really do not get. Right hand touch with knees bend to the side towards the floor and lift upwards towards the left. Alternate on both sides. If done correctly, it should look like you are swinging an ax chopping. But like I said if done correctly but of course mine look nothing at all like that.
10. **Shoulder Tap Plank** – **35s** – plank and tap hand on opposite sides. Right hand taps Left shoulder and Left Hand taps Right shoulder.
11. **Frog Tuck Squat** – **35s** – we did a simpler version. This is like Burpees but when jumping in front, both legs must be at the side of your hands.
12. **Russian Twist** – **35s** – balance on your glutes, lift both legs up mid way and body upright, twist to the right and left and must be done slowly to be effective.
13. **V-Tuck** – **35s** – this is done with sitting, lifting your legs up, extending your legs forward and bringing back towards your chest and as you are doing this, move your body also. This is a clam shell – opening and closing.

14. **V-Tuck Hold – 35s** – this is done the same as above position but just hold, not sure if this is tougher or moving legs are tougher.
15. **Sit-up Toe Tap** – lift both of your legs straight up to the air and start crunching while your hands reach the toe.
16. **Warrior Plank** – start with Full Plank and slowly place your elbow down alternatively and back to the full plank.

Notes:

This was a good workout as there are combinations of different moves which make it interesting plus at the same time, when you are tired, it's a kind of distraction and before you know it, you have done so much just for an hour! Good mind diversion.

Sweat - 11ml

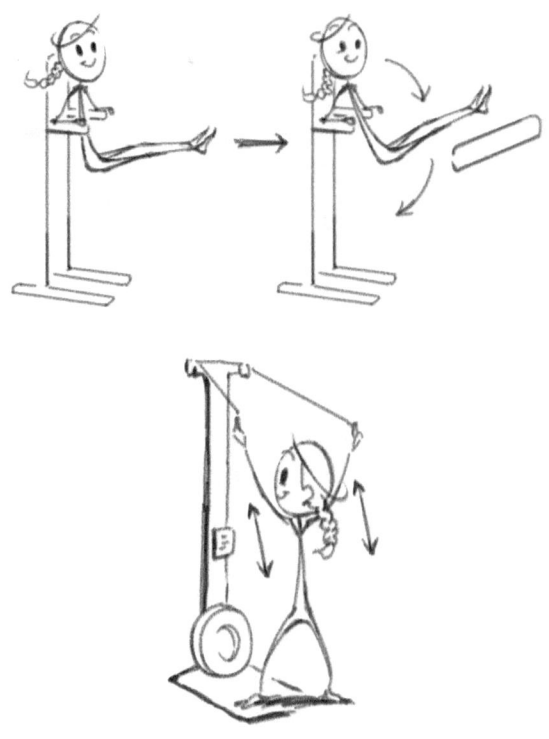

Sweat Session: Crossfit

Mr. Trainer – Let me introduce you to Crossfit, you may know about it already but knowing and doing it are two different worlds....

Lil' Student – This is one of those that when you see people doing it you will go like ooohhhhhh... wahhhhhhh.... I want to do that or I want to be like that... but doing it you will end up... ohhhhhh noooooo... what is all this???

1. **Assault Bike – 30s** – and you need to cycle till you hear the fan sound that would mean, yes you are fine, and plus the louder it is the more wind you will get.

   Burpees – 30s – yes by now you should start accepting this as one of your best friends, might as well like it.

   Mr. Trainer – burpees is the only exercise that makes her tired and she loves it... (not sure when I ever said this ya... so not true till today... still do not like Burpees).

2. **Military Press – 30s** – need to do this continuously for 6 mins x 3 sets (yes there is no typo... it is 6 mins non-stop as 1 set). The longest ever 6 mins in my life....

3. **Skierg – 20 reps x 3 sets** – this machine is like skiing actions with your hands above and pull all the way down and this machine also makes a sound "swoosssssssssshhhhh" and again the louder the better... means you are strong... not much sound means... work harder....

   Mr. Trainer – she did well with good technique. And there are Games on the machine... some kind of fishing game (who wants to even look at a game when you are already dying).

4. **Dumbbell Snatches – 15 reps x 3 sets**
5. **Dumbbell Deadlift – 15 reps x 3 sets**
6. **Dumbbell Push Press – 15 reps x 3 sets**
7. **Dumbbell High Pull – 15 reps x 3 sets** – explosively raise the dumbbells as high as you can, making sure the elbow is pointed high.

   Mr. Trainer – for Dumbbell high pull you need to explosively raise the dumbbell till elbow pointed high. Deadlift is very good.... Shoulders still not very strong but soon will make her weak point become strong....

8. **Ball Slam + Burpees – 10 reps x 3 sets**
9. **Hanging Leg Raises – 10 reps x 3 sets** – this is done on the Monkey Bar but this round do not worry as my legs are in front (so no chance of kicking Mr. Trainer). He was very safe for this exercise….

   Mr. Trainer – she can do leg raises but not with straight legs. Still need to tuck in but slowly she will get there…. But of course I will…

10. **Double Kettlebell Hold – (8kgs) x 2 x 2 sets** – this is done with just holding 2 Kettlebells at your chest level with your elbow tucked in… sounds pretty simple.

    Mr. Trainer – purpose of doing this is to expand the lungs to improve breathing. Same concept like "swimming".

11. **Semi Circle Leg Raise – 10 reps x 3 sets** – you raise your legs while Mr. Trainer holds a Tube and your legs need to raise over the Tube and cannot touch the Tube.

    Mr. Trainer – core is improving but maybe fatigue starts up, as counts go by the legs slowly going down…

    Serious Note: I had to do "Ketuk Ketampi" x 4 times because my legs touched the Tube. What is "Ketuk Ketampi" – please Google it… this is not funny as I did this in front of people in the Gym ya….

Notes:

Crossfit is very intense but it is very satisfying when you see what you have done and learned so many different exercises in just an hour. Dying is a given no need to mention for every workout… just at what level….

Sweat - 12ml

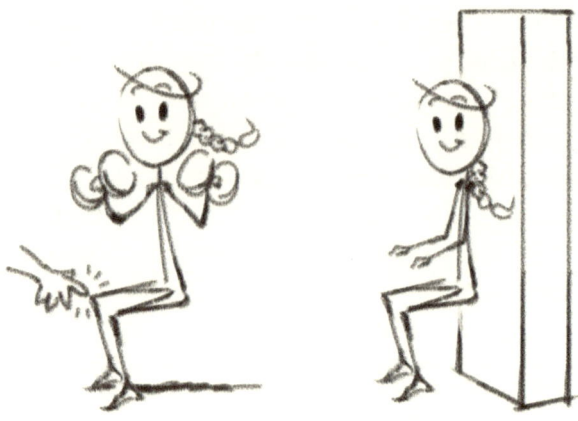

Sweat Session: Leg Day

Mr. Trainer – There is a saying that you control your Legs today but 2 days later your Legs will control your world…. Let's find out what this means.

Lil' Student – Ok yes I totally agree with the above statement as I have shared my moments of legs controlling my life but after a while when you start to see your legs getting into shape – it is just satisfying and it is so so worth it, trust me… (do you believe me???) hahaha…. One of my goals for legs are – the East and the West of the inner quads should never be friends though they literally do see each other everyday and live next to each other, but they should never be friends.

1. **Bicycle** – 5 mins warm up to get the heart pumping. Heart rate was 160.

2. **Leg Extension Machine** – (7.5kg) x 12 x 3 sets – (no need to wonder any more as minimal sets are set at 3 ya)…. Did this well…
   Mr. Trainer – can see defined muscles, legs are getting stronger.

3. **Wall Sit** – **15s x 3 sets** – you lean on a wall and sit - imagine there is a chair and hold for a specific time in this case it's 15s. Need finger assistance getting up… not sure if sitting and holding is harder or getting up… normally after 2nd set, confirm will need finger assistance to get up.

4. **Jumping Jacks – 30s**

5. **Piston Squat (TRX)** – **x 15 x 3 sets** – ok have done this in TRX class but… why is it always so much harder when it's done with Mr. Trainer?? Because it's done with the correct technique and if done correctly - omg feel the burn…. This move with 1 leg lifted up and you squat up and down.

6. **Plank to Pike**

7. **Semi Circle Leg Raises** – (with Mr. Trainer's favourite Pipe again…) lift both legs and circle around the pipe and it's not my imagination and I am not dizzy ya… the Pipe tends to get higher and higher as we progress from 1st set – 2nd set – 3rd set. Now this is when the argument will start about how low or high the Pipe is but learned my lesson the hard way – don't bother, don't waste your breath as you will always lose the battle and still have to finish your set.

8. **Leg Extension Machine** – **(12.5kg) x 12 x 3 sets** – to develop the "pocket" muscles at the side… ya and pocket for me to carry my water tumbler??? Or my towel??

9. **Jump Squat** – **10 x 3 sets**
   Mr. Trainer – improved in terms of landing (not like a Hippo), slowly progressing.

10. **TRX Jump Squat – 10 x 3 sets** – learned the proper way to do this, when you jump your hands on straps you must push down and not grab the strap and keep jumping.

Mr. Trainer – new concept, new technique and now she can teach everyone from making the same mistake (if I still remember it in the next class…).

Sweat - 13ml

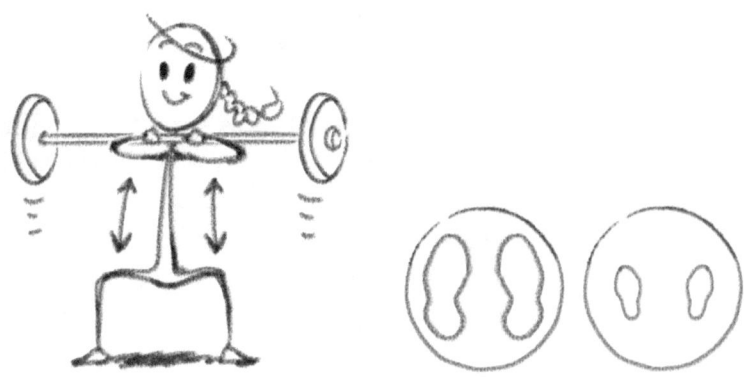

Sweat Session: HIIT (High Intensity Interval Training)

Mr. Trainer – Lil' Student – let's get a bit next level today.

Lil' Student – The name says it all right… well let's see where I will end up… and everything is 45s.

1. **Squat Press – (10kg) x 45s**
   Mr. Trainer – legs are still shaking but getting stronger everyday.
2. **KettleBell Deadlift – (8kg) x 45s**
   Mr. Trainer – posture and technique well performed but lost track when "Lil' Student" gets tired.
3. **Burpees – 45s** – told you that this will be one of your best friends hahaha.
4. **Dumbbell Skierg Swing – (3kg) x 45s** – same movement as the Skierg machine but need lots of power to control the movement using dumbbell.

5. **Dumbbell Bent Over Row** – **(3kg) x 45s** – now anything to do with "Row" please take note as this is another killer move.

   Mr. Trainer – needs improvement on technique so that it will really target the muscle part… (so what are you saying?? That I did all 45s for nothing and no muscles were worked on???).

6. **Dumbbell Split Jerk** – **(3kg) x 45s** – jerk movements are another hard-to-do as this is coordination with hands and legs, can only function with max 2 limbs at the same time, anything more it will all go hay-wire – which hand goes where and which leg supposed to go where??? First time doing this and you can imagine what happened – not very much was done and not done properly. It is done with hands up holding dumbbells and as your hands go down, your legs need to shuffle back and forth concurrently…

7. **Dumbbell Squat** – **(3kg) x 45s** – make sure knees are not exceeding toes. Still need pointers till now as Mr. Trainer still needs to put his fingers to ensure my knees do not exceed the toe.

8. **Dumbbell Lunges** – **(3kg) x 45s** – doing good but got distracted by an inappropriate scenario of a couple nearby… 18SX cannot be revealed here.

9. **Bosu Squats** – did well on balancing myself on the Bosu while squatting but legs were shaking like "Pepper Shaker". Challenged Mr. Trainer to do this. But of course he did it effortlessly and with no "shaking" effects at all.

   My theory – Mr. Trainer your feet are so much bigger and wider so of course you can cover the base more which equals to more stability right? Vs my tiny penguin feet…

Sweat - 14ml

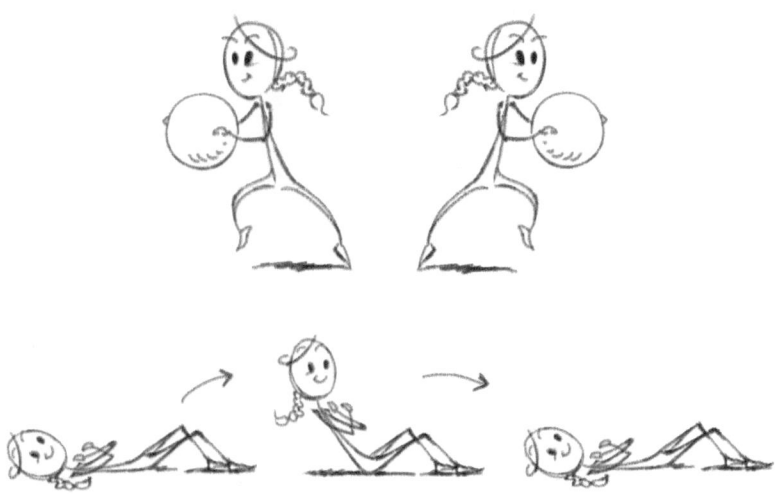

Sweat Session: Full Body (30seconds day)

Mr. Trainer – Today we will do a full body workout.

Lil' Student – The good thing about full body workout is that we do not get bored as there are variances but the bad thing is that when the soreness hits, it's also FULL BODY in pain.

1. **Squat – 16 reps, 15 reps, 16 reps x 30s each** – still under the finger supervision of knees not exceeding toes… (depending on individual some are allowed to slightly exceed due to body posture as long as you don't feel any tension on your knees). Angles matter: for those who have injuries it will be done differently.
Mr. Trainer – movement was okay, just a bit stiff on calves and ankles.

2. **Biceps Curl – 20 reps, 18 reps, 19 reps x 30s each** – always focus on isolation and concentric movement.

   Mr. Trainer – lines are showing. GOOD SIGN (muscles growing everyday)!!

3. **Shoulder Press – 15 reps, 13 reps, 12 reps x 30s each**

   Mr. Trainer – need to strengthen shoulder muscles + improve muscle stabilization right and left by playing around with the tempo (slow pace).

4. **High Knees – 30s** – sweat starts flowing, in other words waterworks start....

   Mr. Trainer – superb movement that tires her easily but still manageable.

5. **Jumping Jacks – 30s** – love doing Jumping Jacks (only when it's not more than 30s) and by far the only move that I can do nicely and Mr. Trainer is silent, which means I'm doing it right.

   Mr. Trainer – cardio movement to increase endurance phase and improve coordination.

6. **Static Jump – 30s** – this is done by touching the floor and jumping up and repeating. Sweat increases drastically now.

   Mr. Trainer – knees' joints are strong with soft landing (finally...) can control muscle execution during jumping.

7. **Lunges with Holding Medicine Ball – 4 reps each side x 3 sets** – this move is done with holding the ball above your head while you do lunges on both legs, sounds easy but not easy at all. Lunges are hard enough, try balancing the ball while doing it... this should be considered as 2 moves ya....

   Mr. Trainer – balancing needs to be improved by developing leg sensitivity and muscle control...

8. **Step In Out – 30s** – stand with one foot on each

side of the Stepper and jump on Stepper, jump again to the sides of the Stepper.

Mr. Trainer – accessory movement to increase heart rate to sustain.

9. **Mountain Climber – 30s**

Mr. Trainer – good because it contracts abs. Ankle mobility needs to improve so she can run faster.

10. **Glutes Raises – 8 reps x 30s x 2 sets**

Mr. Trainer – awesome workout to build up and reshape glutes and sharpen the looks of hamstrings (hmm… hamstrings also needs to have "The Look").

Sweat - 15ml

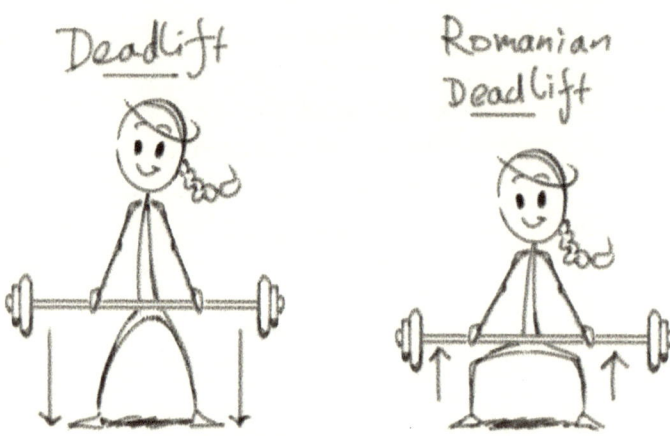

Sweat Session: Leg Day (yes again...)

Mr. Trainer – Yes before we even realized it, it's Leg Day again.

Lil' Student – Leg Day is still a day that I drag myself to the Gym as I can already feel the soreness even before I reach the GYM... but I still have to do it...

1. **Leg Extension – (17.5kg) 12 reps x 3 sets**
   Mr. Trainer – muscles are defined, good work on maintaining tempo and strength on legs are improving.
2. **Hamstring Curls – (12.5kg) x 12 reps x 3 sets –**
   this is done while laying on your tummy and hook your ankles to the cushioned part of the bench

and start to lift till the cushioned part touches your hamstring or glutes.

Mr. Trainer – sharp hamstrings, need to focus more on the upper part of hamstrings (head) which is located right under glutes (and I thought hamstrings are your calves, but I guess not, it's right up to your glutes).

3. **Leg Press – (5kg) x 8 reps x 3 sets, (12.5kg) x 12 reps x 3 sets** – you put both feet on the pad of the machine, press and as you press your body will go up and down. Lots of work on the Quads and Glutes… normally this is the one that will give me super painful sorenesss…

   Mr. Trainer – focuses more on Hip Flexor (Quads/ Hamstrings/Glutes) and good to build up testosterone levels for females. Well performed and worked on tempo (hmmm… women need testosterone??? It seems we do and it helps with growth, maintaining women's reproductive tissues and bone mass).

4. **Reverse Lunges – 10 reps each side x 3 sets** – not my favourite move.

   Mr. Trainer – legs are slightly tight on the adductors (inner thigh) because knees tend to move inward. Need to stretch and do activation movement on the abductors (outer thigh).

5. **Back Squats – Barbell (12.5kg) x 10 reps x 3 sets**
   Mr. Trainer – movement is good. Ankle mobility is improving. Range of motion getting bigger.

6. **Romanian Deadlift – (12.5kg) x 10 reps x 3 sets** – you lower the Barbell lowest to your shin and lift up again – do not touch the ground. Focus totally on the hamstring, best for developing tail hamstrings.

Notes:

Finisher was TRX Jump Squat – this is not a part of the above exercise but just an add-on based on Mr. Trainer's mood. Shall we do one more??? Sureee why not… this is normally called a "play around session".

Sweat - 16ml

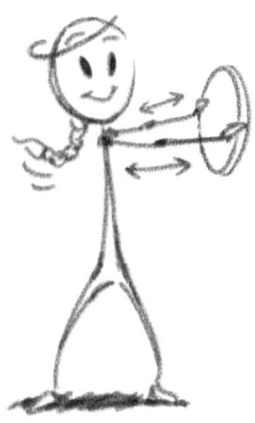

Sweat Session: Shoulder Day

Mr. Trainer – Today is all about Push and Press.

Lil' Student – Shoulder Day seems easy but at times I still struggle to finish the sets. And normally after a Shoulder Day, I cannot even wipe my back with the towel and have to leave it to air dry… why? Because I cannot lift my arms and don't even mention removing a sports bra – I will need to bend over. Yes it is quite funny….

1. **Chest Press Machine – (10kg) x 12 reps x 3 sets**
   Mr. Trainer – works more on the upper chest. Benefit of doing this is to lift up the chest and develop good posture – hmmmm… what does this mean? **(Working your chest will strengthen your pectoral muscles and possibly give your breasts a more lifted appearance).**

2. **Hindu Press – (2.5kg) x 10 reps x 3 sets**
   Mr. Trainer – accessory work right after chest press machine to trigger the muscles and maintain contraction.
3. **Incline Dumbbell Chest Press – (4kg) x 10 reps x 3 sets**
   Mr. Trainer – body symmetry, both sides need to have the same force execution for best results (obviously mine is not as my left side has less strength).
4. **Incline Dumbbell Fly – (4kg) x 10 reps x 3 sets**
   Mr. Trainer – to get rid of excessive fat at the side of the chest and to develop chest shape. Factors that can contribute is chest lift.
5. **Incline Dumbbell Close Grip – (4kg) x 10 reps x 3 sets**
   Mr. Trainer – best for upper chest muscle.

Notes:

Today's session seems like a short session but trust me it was not – in the next 2 days my arms will hurt and have limited functionality.

Sweat - 17ml

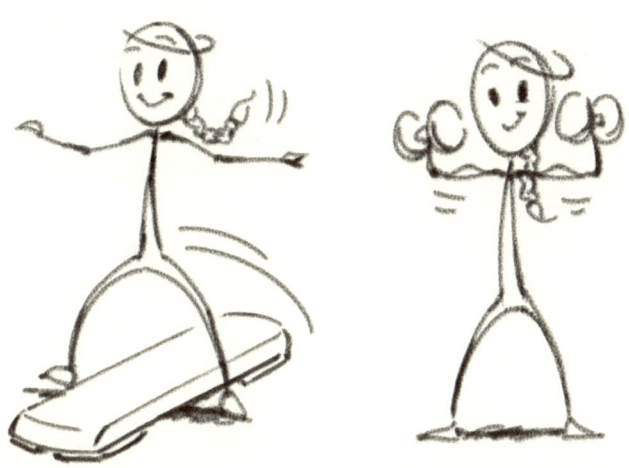

Sweat Session: Full Body

Mr. Trainer – Combination.

1. **Cycling – warm up**
    Mr. Trainer – great move for warming up and for interval training. Quads muscles are involved during this movement as the faster you go, you feel it more on your quads.
2. **Deadlift – (15kg) x 10 reps x 3 sets** – did this and ended with a Big Smile.
    Mr. Trainer – movement is getting better and the hamstring is not as stiff as before. Lower back getting stronger and it is a good sign because your spine is aligned and muscle tissues are well developed.
3. **Burpees – 6 reps** – side by side – this is done by

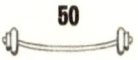

doing 1 burpee move and jump over a Barbell and another burpee on the other side.

Mr. Trainer – your burpees are getting better and you can go more than 50 reps already! It's just a matter of endurance and stamina (ya, right, if it's 50 reps it's not longer Burpees, it's Deadpees ya).

4. **Thread the needle (ViPR) (8kg)** – this is the Pipe again where you hold it and swing it under your legs and up above your head. I was more concerned about not hitting my head.

   Mr. Trainer – new movement for you but as I mentioned above that your back is strong so the movement is smooth. Just the ViPR might be slightly heavy for you to turn but it's okay. GOOD JOB!! E for Excellent!!!

5. **Barbell Front Squat – (10kg) x 8 reps x 3 sets** – rest Barbell with your arms and hold it against your chest and lift your elbows up to balance it and if your elbows are not up the Bar will slip. And start squatting....

   Mr. Trainer – squat improved a lot due to tremendous hours spent training and torturing sessions, but hips are slightly tight but all is well. Oooh... the bar is slipping off... Mr. Trainer – "Lil' Student just lift your elbows." (jeeezzzz... thanks for your help...).

Notes:

Based on the good job done I believe I have improved quite a bit and am feeling more confident. At this stage Mr. Trainer does not assist much anymore but just merely stand there and tell me how to do it vs earlier days, he will assist with his fingers tips. Guess I'm getting stronger already.

Sweat - 18ml

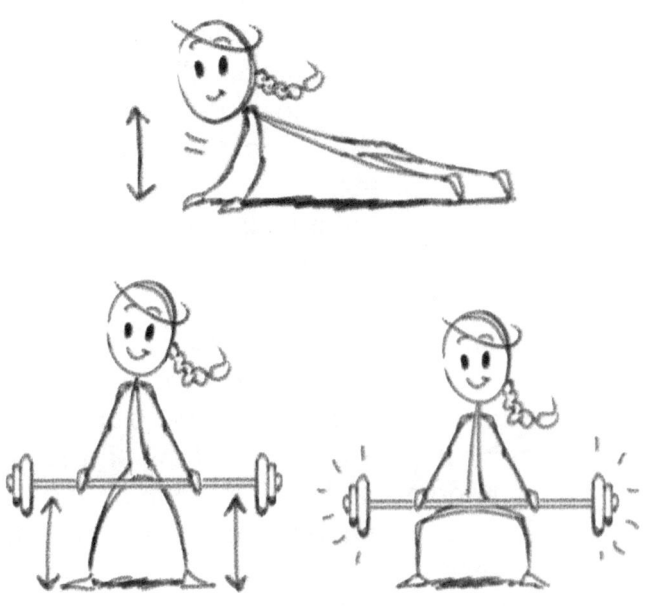

Sweat Session: Strength

Mr. Trainer – More fun coming up….

Lil' Student – Strength days can be super fun as we will do lots of different exercises but at the same time it is super tiring too.

1. **Push-up (10 reps) + Sumo Deadlift (15kg) x (10 reps) x 3 sets** – still cannot really do full push-ups. Push-ups combo with sumo deadlift as the first set of exercise really felt like it's the end of the session. Energy level just went from 100% to 20%. How to make it through the next hour….

Mr. Trainer – still needs to work on push-ups in terms of upper body strength. Sumo deadlift movement is perfect as your major muscle activation is more on the lower body. This is too easy for you so added weights… (but I still did well!).

2. **Pull Up with Resistant Band** – Monkey Bar – this is super fun – you hang yourself on the Monkey Bar with a Resistant Band and do pull ups. Baby level of pull ups I'm guessing.

Scenario 1 – what if I fall as the Resistant Band is not that wide ya, will Mr. Trainer be able to dive and save me in time?

Scenario 2 – what if I fall and Mr. Trainer does not make it but I fall on him!!! Thinking about which scenario will work better – back up plan - we always must have a back up plan, right, and at the same time trying not to knock my chin on the Bar while pulling up. I think I worked on my brain muscles more than my body muscles for this move.

Mr. Trainer – ok Bye Lil' Student… (and I was left hanging on that Monkey Bar). Hellooo…

3. **Lat Pull Down – (20.5kg) x 10 reps + Squat x 10 reps x 3 sets**

Mr. Trainer – develop latissimus dorsi or wings. Now everyone can fly from here…. Wings developed well and back muscles are defined (if only I can see my back, and this is when Mr. Trainer will take videos to show me my Wings!!!).

4. **Hamstring Curl – (14kg) x 10 reps x 3 sets**

Mr. Trainer – you really have sharp hamstrings and it makes your lower body look nicer. Hamstrings are connected to your glutes and give your butt (helloo, glutes ya we do not use the word "butt" in the fitness world…) more shape.

5. **Bench Dumbbell Press – (5kg) x 8 reps + Push-up (10 reps) x 3 sets**

   Mr. Trainer – chest muscle activation. Checked. Now you know how to really use your chest muscles. For Push-up, the major target is the chest but at the moment you feel it on your triceps due to your arm strength. Arms strong, upper body strong.

6. **Crawl + Crab Reverse – 6 reps x 3 sets** – done with hand placed behind hips up and crawl. Body facing upward and needs to crawl forward and backward.

   Mr. Trainer – still needs to improve in terms of your flexibility and mobility (yes 2 more out of the 50 weaknesses). Hips need to be mobile in order for you to reach behind when doing crab reserve. Mobility and flexibility are good to improve coordination, speed and agility....

Notes:

As per above, mobility, flexibility is not my forte and I really need more and more work on that.

Sweat - 19ml

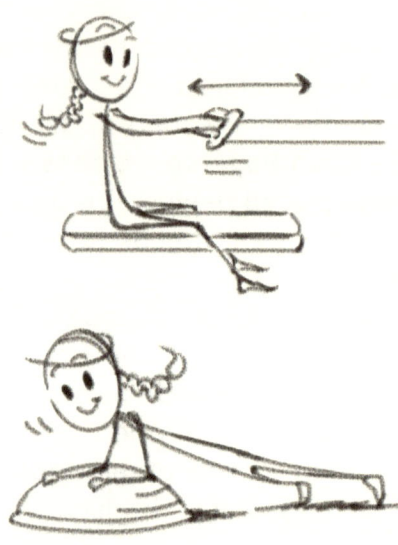

Sweat Session: Back Day

Mr. Trainer – Objective of the Day – to look like HourGlass.

Lil' Student – Back exercise and you will hear a lot of wings being mentioned. I would say this is not that hard as most of the moves are done on machines.

1. **Lat Pull Down Machines – (20.5kg) x 10 reps x 3 sets**

   Mr. Trainer – back is getting stronger and the wings are there. Even Mr. Trainer uses my terms now. The best is when you do it with muscle mind connection. Keep on doing it and you will develop the muscle mind connection within time (yes it does not get any more complicated than this, from proper form, technique, tempo and now mind connection??).

2. **Rowing Machine – (15.5kg) x 12 reps x 3 sets –**
this is a machine with a handle that is connected to a cable, you sit and hold the handle and pull towards your rib.
Mr. Trainer – increase the size of your back or we call it rhomboids. Increase size as in wide body to look like hourglass (hmmm... my body already does look like hourglass... but I'm sure your answer will be – yes but we will need to maintain so please continue...).

3. **Rowing Machine (Wide) – (15.5kg) x 12 reps x 3 sets**
Mr. Trainer – same muscles as above. Attack more on the rhomboid and the teres major of your back to make it more defined.

4. **Rowing Machine – Single Row – (7kg) x 12 reps x 3 sets**
Mr. Trainer – single movement works best on increasing the symmetry of the muscle. Correcting the muscle and bone alignment.

5. **Reverse Fly – (3kg) x 12 reps x 3 sets**
Mr. Trainer – develop muscles behind your armpits (teres minor). So when you wear sleeveless it will look nice and fit.

6. **Leg Raises – 10 reps x 3 sets**
Mr. Trainer – core getting stronger day by day as per the adaptation of the muscles.

7. **Bosu Plank – (New movement) –** balance both hands on Bosu and with plank position and hold, this adds more intensity as well as balance.
Mr. Trainer – body symmetry and best to learn how to control your body. For you, you will see the true potential of your body if you control all of it.

Sweat - 20ml

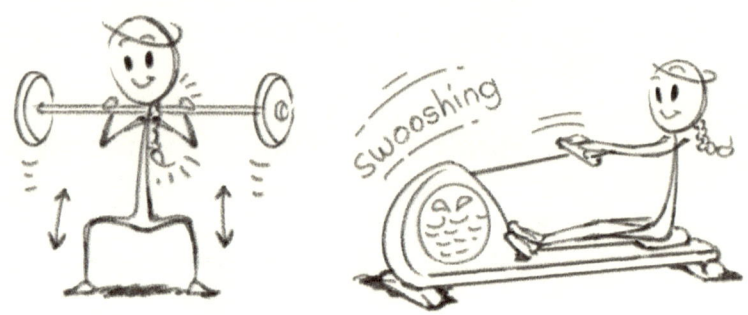

Sweat Session: Strength

Mr. Trainer – Another fun day and we have a new machine today.

Lil' Student – A new machine?? I shall not fear the need to embrace new challenges. Let's do this.

1. **Rowing Machine aka Washing Machine** – this is a machine where it has a Big Circle like a Wheel in front and it's filled with water and you sit with your legs strapped in and you start to pull the handle towards your ribs and as you pull, the Wheel will start to churn and you can literally hear the water swooshing sound. This is either done by seconds or by metres or to reach certain metres by a certain time frame. Mainly to test your endurance.
Mr. Trainer – expressed concern that it took her minutes to strap on her legs, but I strapped her legs within a second (but once you are strapped in, you can't escape anymore).

2. **Barbell Squat – (12kg) x 15 reps x 3 sets** – done with Barbell resting on the back of your shoulder and squat. But there is always a situation here – my Pigtail is stuck!! Mr. Trainer's extra effort will have to make sure Pigtail is moved to the side before I rest the Barbell.

   Mr. Trainer – her legs are getting stronger now as the shaky part is not visible anymore. Body and Torso is not bent forward compared to last time. GOOD IMPROVEMENT AND VERY IMPRESSIVE....

3. **Kettlebell Reverse Lunges – (8kg) x 16 reps x 3 sets**

   Mr. Trainer – needs to learn to bring her legs further behind. There is a difference between Lunges and Split Squats. Lunges push your legs all the way behind while Split Squats just maintain 90°.

4. **Dumbbell Alternate Shoulder Press – (5kg) x 12 reps x 3 sets**

   Mr. Trainer – due to lack of shoulder mobility, can see it's not going straight up but towards outward. But in terms of strength yes she really improved a lot.

5. **Dumbbell Lateral Raises – (4kg) x 10 reps x 3 sets** – holding dumbbell and lifting your arms on the sides.

   Mr. Trainer – even though shoulders are not mobile but can see her shoulders getting more defined. Getting wide and she looks really fit from behind (only from behind??? We need to look fit – 360° ya).

6. **Dumbbell Military Press – (6kg) x 10 reps x 3 sets**

   Mr. Trainer – superb movement, managed to carry it but still needs assistance. Overall I can see the strength in her is really POWER!! Superb Progress!

7. **Leg Raises – 10 reps x 3 sets**
   Mr. Trainer – core getting stronger day by day. Seems like leg raises don't work for her anymore. It's my job to change them (there is just no way to cheat my way – once I have adapted to a move – need to level up already).

8. **Dumbbell Hammer Curl – (4kg) x 10 reps x 3 sets** – same as bicep curls but instead of being done at the sides, this is done with both hands in front and elbow does not move. Stick the elbow to your body.
   Mr. Trainer – building the muscles on your biceps but still need to focus more on the contraction part and put more attention on not moving your elbows.

9. **Tricep Push Down – (32.5kg) x 15 reps x 3 sets** – you sit on this machine and push down with your triceps.

Sweat - 21ml

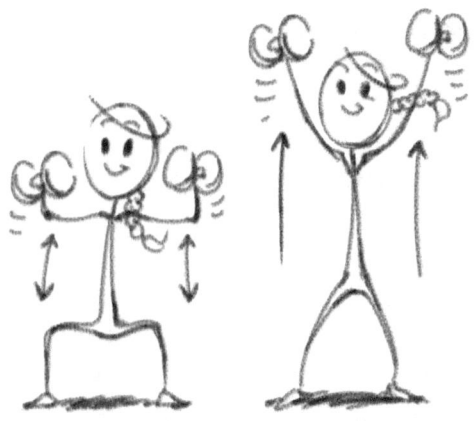

Sweat Session: Full Body - Strength

Mr. Trainer – How are you today?? (with a Smile as always)

Lil' Student – Fine but just here and there is sore… not like anyone is even listening ya….

1. **Dumbbell Thruster – (6kg) x 10 reps x 3 sets –** hold dumbbells and squat. When you come up, you raise both hands above your head.
   Mr. Trainer – pelvic movement needs to improve. Overall movement is good, just need to train more on pelvic push explosions (this sounds so scary right…). Pelvic movement is minor and the major part is movement on the shoulder.
2. **Kettlebell Deadlift – (6kg) x 10 reps x 3 sets** – place the kettlebell at the side of your each leg and lift them up like doing normal deadlift movement.

3. **Kettlebell Rotate** – **(8kg) x 10 reps x 3 sets** – this movement is to check shoulder mobility.
Mr. Trainer – mobility is very good because she managed to do it with 8kg rotation.

4. **Barbell Thruster** – **(6kg) x 10 reps x 3 sets** – squat with Barbell and when you go up you need to push the barbell overhead.
Mr. Trainer – getting better everyday for squat movement but when she feels tired, all movements are forgotten....

5. **Push Up** – **45s**
Mr. Trainer – tricep power is developing and can say she is very strong now. Push-up 45s is not something easy but yet she managed to complete (could it be that his watch was wrong? Are you sure I did 45s?).

6. **V Crunch** – **45s (New Move)** – lie down with hands extended over your head. As you lift your hands up, you lift your legs above the floor too – must do together.
Mr. Trainer – stiff on hip flexor and this makes it hard to lift legs. Overall for a first timer, this is good enough.

7. **Assault Bike** – **45s**
Mr. Trainer – best to train endurance. Need to improve. Slowly but surely and at one point this will be a warm up movement (yes you are so right as now this is one of my warm up movements already).

Notes:

As Mr. Trainer always says for certain movements that it will one day be my warm up move, and yet at that time, I just laugh it off with a – ya right... but honestly I do believe him now as I can do that already.

Sweat - 22ml

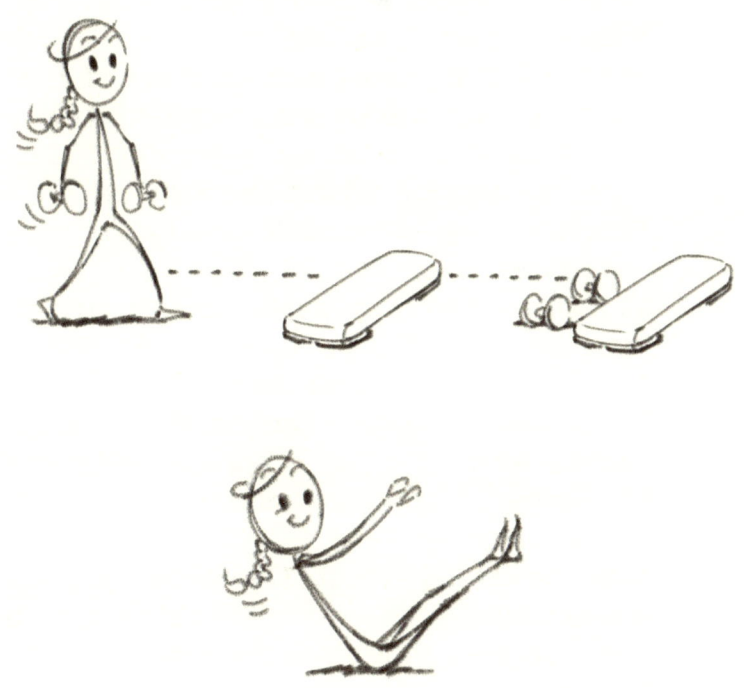

Sweat Session – Crossfit Again

Mr. Trainer – We will be doing a more interesting crossfit today.

Lil' Student – Ooh no… hope I will be still intact after this training.

1. **Dumbbell Carry + FlipBoard – (10kg) 5 in 1 ladder** – you carry the dumbbell and walk over the Step Board and place dumbbell down and turn around, pick up the Step Board, place it in front

and carry the dumbbell by walking over the Step Board again. Repeat for 5 times and you will reach the finishing line.

Mr. Trainer – check her strength and laziness (what does this mean?? Laziness???). If she is lazy she won't pick up the Step Board and move it forward but she proved to everyone she can and a person who does not give up easily (hmmm.... Didn't think I had a choice not to follow the rules...).

2. **Thruster – (6kg) – Dumbbell** – squat with dumbell and lift over head.

   Mr. Trainer – a bit tough as she needs to push and press the weight of 6kg on each hand. Regress it to only 1 dumbbell with both hands.

3. **Wood Chop – (6kg) – Dumbbell** – develop a stronger core.

   Mr. Trainer – did great and maintained the momentum.

4. **Side Leg Lateral – (6kg) – Dumbbell** – you stand and lean shoulder against the wall but feet must be away from the wall. Lift the outer leg while holding the dumbbell.

   Mr. Trainer – feel more on lower glutes and abductors. Good exercise to tone up legs. She can't lift that high due to the tightness of the IT band.

5. **Burpees, burpees and burpees...**

   Mr. Trainer – best exercise for her and it's her favourite movement as she can count the droplets of her sweat.

6. **Squat + Arnold Press** – coordination movement (but of course it was all over the place).

   Mr. Trainer – normal squat and press. Targets quads and shoulders.

7. **Skierg – 30s + Slam Ball – (8kg)** – to check endurance and speed.

Mr. Trainer – as she goes faster the skierg will produce a louder spin sound. The spinning sound is getting louder as she knows how to execute the force at a certain angle… (finally I got it!).

8. **Inchworm and Crab Touch Toe** – looks like a worm walking but it's human.
   Mr. Trainer – targets hamstring and core. Balancing is off but managed to control so she didn't fall down.

9. **V Crunch** – requires total abs strength. Need to lift my body and arms higher.

Notes:

Sometimes the list of moves seems like less but do not be fooled, when it's a shorter list of moves, it means higher reps and harder or it could be 1 move + another move means each exercise has 2 in 1.

Sweat - 23ml

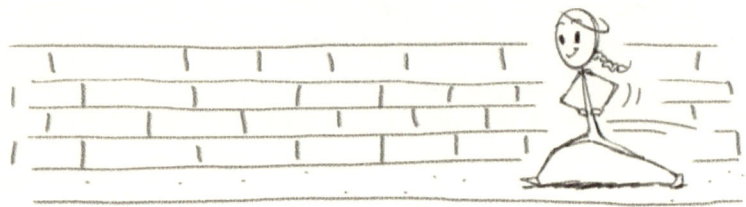

Sweat Session – Leg Day Again and Again

Mr. Trainer – Hello… how are you today?

Lil' Student – Mr. Trainer will always sound and look more cheerful on dying days. You do know that you do not fool me that easily anymore as I have a list of your smile types… and what it means.

1. **Leg Press – (25kg) x 10 reps x 3 sets** – both legs on the machines and start pushing up and down.
   Mr. Trainer – do it like a boss as if there is no feel. Legs are getting stronger, more muscles developing.
2. **Single Leg Press – (7.5kg) x 8 reps x 3 sets** –
   same as above but with only 1 leg and the other leg remaining straight, always a dying move and it makes your glutes feel like something is going to snap.
   Mr. Trainer – this movement is her enemy as it makes her glutes sore for days. But a good sacrifice because she will have nice glutes to show off. No Pain, No Gain.

3. **Hamstring Curl – (15.5kg) x 10 reps x 3 sets**
   Mr. Trainer – hamstrings are getting sharper and can see definition. New hamstring looks perfect on her.
   Actual scenario – hamstring was pulling so much it felt like cramping. Had to stop and Mr. Trainer had to massage my calves, to ease it….

4. **Walking Lunges** – for all "newbies" this is 1 move that we can't get away with and it's just a matter of time when you will need to do it. The length of the Gym hallway where I did this was like walking "The Great Wall of China"… Mr. Trainer's voice in the background "Legs more back and wider"… the sound effect that lingers all the way… and there is no mute button.

5. **Seated Hamstring Curls – (21kg) x 8 reps x 3 sets** – done on a machine that makes me feel like a "sandwich"… why? It clamps your legs/ankles and now that you are clamped in, you can't escape and the only way out is to finish the set.
   Mr. Trainer – same as lying hamstring curl, targets hamstrings to make it more defined.

6. **Good Morning – (12.5kg)** – hamstring movement and can be done every day when you wake up. Good for blood flow in the body.

7. **Glutes Bridge – (6.25kg & 11.25kg) x 10 reps x 3 sets** – done with this cable that is attached to 2 balls at the end. Stand with legs apart with cable in between your legs and pull the cable outwards.
   Mr. Trainer – requires her pelvis to go forward and squeeze her glutes really hard. Great movement for good looking glutes… (oh boy today it's all about Glutes and Hamstrings…).

8. **Sit-up Benches – 10 reps x 3 sets** – lie on the bench and hold the handle above your head and

start raising your legs.

Mr. Trainer – core is getting stronger and stronger. Very proud of her. Still remember how the first time she used her core and it was the hardest thing to do on earth.

9. **V Crunch – 10 reps x 3 sets**

Mr. Trainer – better this round as she can lift her body higher.

Sweat - 24ml

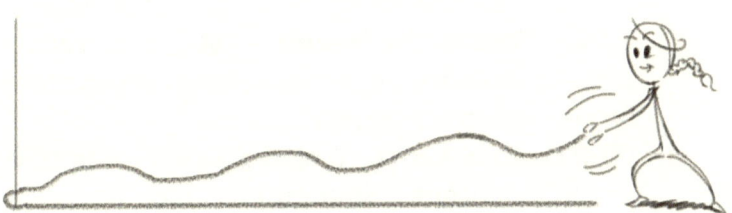

Sweat Session – Battle Rope is BACK!!!

Mr. Trainer – Ready to whip some ropes?!

Lil' Student – Guess my break-in plan did not happen as we are back with the Rope.

1. **Battling Rope – 30s** – high intensity workout. Burns more calories than cycling.
   Mr. Trainer – first try she did it with shoulder and got better by only moving her hands (elbow to forearm).
2. **Rope + Slam Ball – 30s x 5 reps** – rope is a very good movement to strengthen the upper body. Toning up is very effective and adding Slam Ball will make it a good and intense combination.
3. **Rope + Push Up – 30s x 5 reps x 3 sets**
   Mr. Trainer – very good as she really goes all the way out for this movement. Rope requires tricep movement and plus push up will make her tricep really start to burn.

4. **Rope One hand – 15s x 5 reps x 3sets** – more towards stabilisation and great core movement.
   Mr. Trainer – very good core but needs to practise as rope waves are at the front line and the back line just stays silent waiting for her to lift them up.
5. **ViPR – Thread the Needle – (8kg) x 10 reps x 3 sets** – endurance movement, makes coordination better and attacks quadriceps too.
6. **ViPR Lunges Assist – 6 reps x 3 sets** – Hamstrings and Quadriceps. Strengthens hip flexor and stability.
   Mr. Trainer – movement is good, need to improve balance maybe due to weakened knees.

Notes:

Notice the list seems short but intensity is very high. This is what we mean by – **IT'S NOT HOW MUCH YOU DO BUT MORE OF WHAT YOU DO**.

Sweat - 25ml

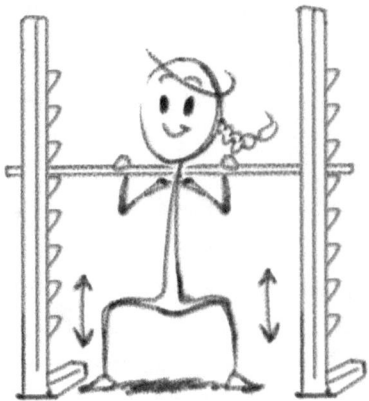

Sweat Session – Full Body - Compound

Mr. Trainer – Today we will do a combination of full body.

Lil' Student – By now even though the reps are not high but intensity definitely has increased and this can be in terms of variance of workout or heavier weights.

1. **Deadlift – (37.5kg) x 10 reps x 3 sets –** good exercise for the postural chain. Improve spine strength and alignment.
   Mr. Trainer – she did great because 37.5kg is not a small weight for a woman. Well Done!
2. **Assisted Pull Up – (20kg) x 10 reps x 3 sets –** this is an assisted machine where you kneel on an elevated pad with both hands on the handle above and start to pull yourself up. This machine works the other way round, the heavier the weight – the easier it is, and the lighter the weight – the harder it is.

Mr. Trainer – now she can fly as she really developed her back well and this movement is really good for making the back shredded.

3. **03. Smith Machine Squat – (27.5kg) x 10 reps x 3 sets** – even though it's assisted but I still feel the struggle especially 2nd set onwards and that's when my Quads will start to burn and it's very hard to stand up.

   Mr. Trainer – her favourite movement which attacks more than Quads and if go lower can attack glutes as well (I think going down is not a problem but the lower you go the harder it is to get up).

4. **Rowing Machine (washing machine) – (1m)** – accessory movement for endurance part. Add on or as interval exercise which is a great combination with compound movement.

5. **Chest Press Machine – (12.5kg) x 10 reps x 3 sets** – this movement is still a struggle as push movement is still not very strong.

   Mr. Trainer – push movement getting there and muscle contraction is real. Really focus on targeted muscle – which is really good.

6. **Plank (1m 5s/1m/1m)** – this is done based on 3 sets and each set is how long you can hold the Plank. Best done with Netflix.

   Mr. Trainer – easy movement for her as she will do this anytime, anywhere. Her base core is really strong and solid.

Notes:

As I progress with strength (can carry heavier weights), there is also endurance that needs to improve. Being strong you may be able to lift heavier weights but endurance will make you last the whole set.

Sweat - 26ml

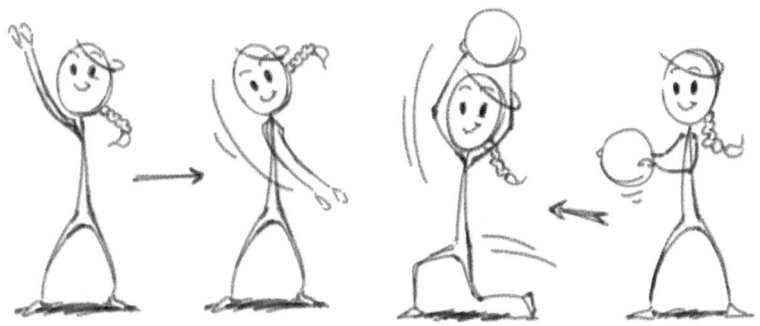

Sweat Session – Upper Body

Mr. Trainer – Are your arms, shoulders and back ready for today?

Lil' Student – As usual none of my body parts are ever ready for any workouts… but I have to always make it look like I'm ready if not Mr. Trainer will do some extreme cardio – to wake me up even before we start and this move will not be part of the workout of the day – it's an extra…

1. **Military Press Dumbbell – (6kg) x 10 reps x 3 sets**
   Mr. Trainer – shoulder movement. She has the strength to push upwards but in terms of stabilizing the arms is not perfect and will go outward without support. Has to be supported on the wrist if not arms will sway out of range.
2. **Arnold Press Dumbbell – (6kg) x 10 reps x 3 sets**
   – Deltoid – a thick triangular muscle covering the shoulder joint. Use for raising the arm away from the body. Great movement for front delt and side delt.

Mr. Trainer – manage to go one flow without stopping but like above – need to improve stabilising this part. Need to train her forearm and wrist so that she controls the upward movement.

3. **Front Shoulder Cable – (5kg) x 10 reps x 3 sets –** front delt attack. Focusing not only on the front delt, it helps in correcting and strengthening the rotator cuff.

   Mr. Trainer – good that she is able to go more than 5 reps but above 5, she starts to get tired.

4. **Cable Curl – (12.5kg) x 10 reps x 3 sets –** focusing more on biceps. Great movement as it provides a big range of motion that helps in muscle growth.

   Mr. Trainer – she is really strong and can call her "Wonder Woman" already.

5. **Rope Tricep Extension – (7.5kg) x 10 reps x 3 sets –** killer movement that makes her triceps sore as this movement requires 100% force from the triceps itself and no assistance.

   Mr. Trainer – getting better but normally if she did this she will definitely say "Cannot la." But she ended up completing the whole set.

6. **Chest Press – (17.5kg) x 10 reps x 3 sets –** again the struggling killer move that I still cannot push on the 3rd set.

   Mr. Trainer – improved in terms of loads vs previous session. Good that she really is developing mind muscle control for her chest pad. Good Job!

Notes:

Upper body movements are not sweaty days but still very tiring and arms will not be 100% functional for the next 2 days.

Sweat - 27ml

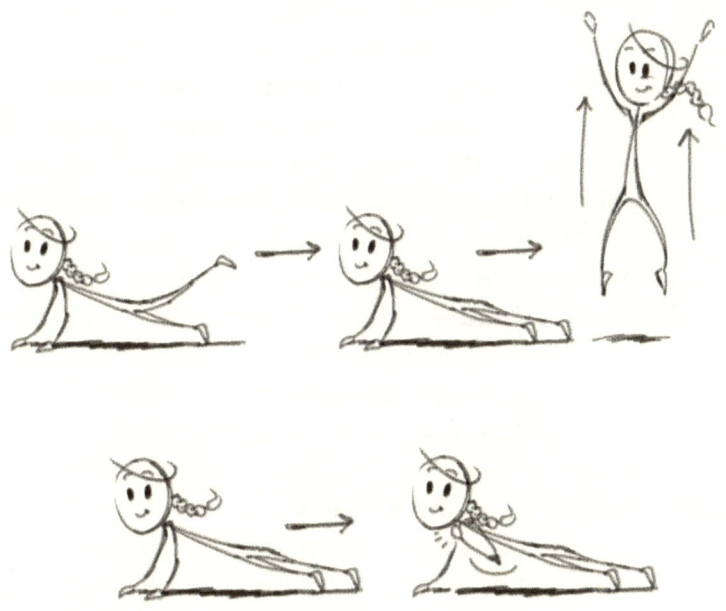

Sweat Session

Mr. Trainer – Here we go again, more rowing and rowing.

Lil' Student – Today is looking like another intense session with Rowing (Washing Machine) always out of breath with just this 1 exercise and it's the first move.

1. **Rowing Machine aka Washing Machine** – 200 metres and did this 3 sets with 56s, 51s, and 50s – looks like the more I do the faster I was…. Best done with singing "Row row row your boat, gently down the stream… as this will distract you from

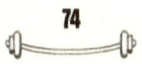

concentrating too much on the numbers on the machine.

Rowing is a great cardiovascular movement. It works on most muscles of your body. Same movement as "kayak" or "water rafting" (both of which I have not done before) well at least with this machine I do not need to get wet due to water but only in my sweat... not sure which is worse.

Mr. Trainer – she really can row with full intensity as she can reach 200m within 1 min. Development of back muscles is much more defined.

2. **Barbell Deadlift + Row – (15kg) x 10 reps x 3 sets** – Deadlift considered full back posture move as the major muscle attack on the hamstring. Add on with barbell row and the resistance will definitely increase.

3. **Burpees + 1 Arm Plank – 8 reps and 20s for Plank – x 3 sets** – endurance based exercise. Great combination. Burpees will pump your heart to the max plus 1 Arm Plank, this is really challenging.

4. **Dumbbell Curl + Reverse Curl – (3kg) x 20 reps x 3 sets** – arms movement basically from biceps all the way to the forearm area.

   Mr. Trainer – if her wrists are weak, this will train them as well. Overall her biceps are really in shape and well defined (and yes, you would think that wrist is the least that needs training right, but actually it does play a role if your wrist is strong, now I know, better mobility).

5. **Dumbbell Curl – (4kg) x 10, 15, 20 reps** – basic curls that really attack the bicep and target at the peak.

   Mr. Trainer – her biceps are well-defined but still needs to work more on the peak, which is basically the top of the biceps.

6. **Lunges – 10 reps x 3 sets** – lower body movement that really challenges your mind when it comes to targeting hamstrings and quads.
   Mr. Trainer – her hip flexor is really strong as she can really stretch out her legs.

7. **Sumo Squat – Barbell (4kg) x 10 reps x 3 sets** – glutes and upper hamstrings target which can really feel the next day. Good movement to bubble up your glutes… (bubble up???).
   Mr. Trainer – her glutes are really nice, just need to touch up… (here only means more work is needed and normally it's not minor work… it's always "touch up" and after it's achieved and then it will be "must maintain" – again continue to do more work).

8. **Side Crunch – 10, 16, 22 reps** – abs based movement where you really feel at the serratus anterior. The more the reps the more you will feel.

Sweat - 28ml

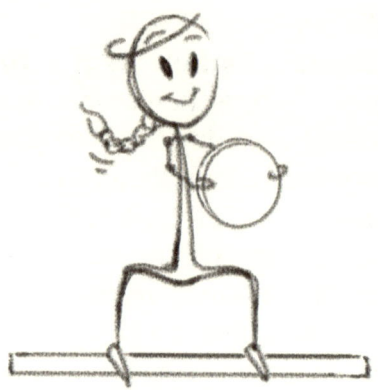

Sweat Session – Mr. Leggy again

Mr. Trainer – Hi did you defrost your Legs in time for today's session?

Lil' Student – Why defrost? As I always told Mr. Trainer that I freeze my muscles and limbs after each session.

1. **Leg Extension – (15.5kg) x 10 reps x 3 sets** – quad development more on saturation or details of the quads and yes this does work ya as now my quads do have a line....
Mr. Trainer – can't really see the saturation as she is wearing tights but can feel the line is there.
2. **Goblet Squats – (5kg) Plate x 10 reps x 3 sets** – Quads dominant, target fully on quads due to the stretch and contraction of the muscle. Heels are on a higher platform and toes on ground and squat while holding the plate instead of dumbbells..

3. **Lying Hamstring Curl – (18.5kg) x 10 reps x 3 sets**
   Mr. Trainer – her hamstring is really sharp. Can cut and slice meat using her hamstrings. Suits her legs as her legs are really nice.
4. **Romanian Deadlift – (9.5kg) x 10 reps x 3 sets –** hamstrings development.
   Mr. Trainer – all good, just need to straighten the back so she can feel the hamstrings more.
5. **Donkey Kick – 10 reps x 3 sets –** Glutes development. Bubbles up glutes and makes it lift up.
6. **Seated Hamstrings Curl – (20kg) x 10 reps x 3 sets –** hamstrings and lower glutes.
   Mr. Trainer – well moved and need to make sure that whenever she pushes down, glutes need to stay on the bench (it's considered "cheating" if your glutes are off the bench, I'm sure you know why Mr. Trainer said that right… ya I cheated and got caught… so whatever reps done that was caught is not counted, do again).
7. **Pauses Squat to Hold Squat – 10 reps x 3 sets**
   Mr. Trainer – can see the shape of her glutes but just need to lift it up (now don't be mistaken here, as our goal is not to have a "brazillian butt" ya).

Notes:

Today is all about Glutes, Glutes and Glutes and it's an effort to even sit after this workout.

Sweating Stops..

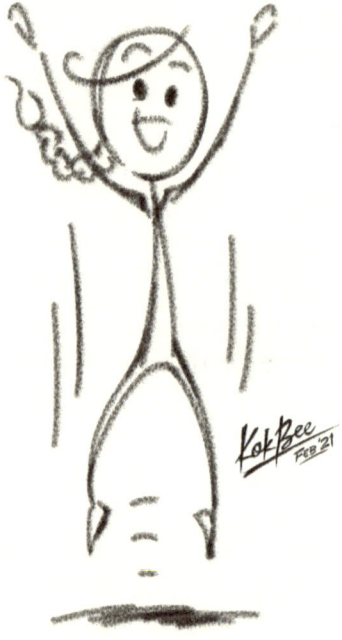

12 months accomplished
(...... or has it really??...... to be contiuned)

Testimonial

See I'm the kind of person that needs facts, figures and visual aid for me to understand and see my progress. Mr. Trainer is to consistently send me progress updates so that it's clear and it's sort of like a motivation tool for me to know how far or much I have progressed. I always love these reports and always look forward to them. Here I would like to thank Mr. Trainer for his dedication and his belief in me that "Nothing is Impossible" and "Age is just a Number". When I heard this Age is just a Number honestly I didn't really believe him, I'm like "right but now I truly believe this 100% as I have proven it to myself that I can do this. Sharing below are his testimonials after 2 months, 4 months and 11 days (yes my Trainer has a lot to do and not just train me in the gym hahaha…).

2 Months - 13 April 2019

No one has made great achievements on the first day. The first sign of a loser is an excuse, champions take full responsibility good or bad for their outcomes. Start grinding and think like a champion. Your Trainer, your boss is not the problem, it's your consistency. Good Job Little Student for putting in such an effort to keep improving yourself. Average is on the left and success on the right, you choose the path.

For someone who did not even know what a Squat is to someone who can handle HIIT. Remember Little Student, I might guide you but you yourself make it happen. Well Done – 100%. Not a single effort of yours will go in vain. You will be rewarded for your pain. Your hard work will bring you a lot of gain.

4 Months and 11 days - 14 June 2019

Little Student, 4 months and 11 days is a long journey for someone who is willing to change their lifestyle. Proud that you are consistent with your training plus all the classes you joined. One of my favourite students that really have that fitness enjoyment kind of spirit. By now I guess you can actually tell yourself how your body condition is. Remember the very first time I met you, I said 1st Phase: Feel, 2nd Phase: See and 3rd Phase: Maintenance.

By now you are already in the 2nd Phase and all the workout is not the beginner kind of workout anymore. Really appreciate that you note down all the things you've learned from me. As well as the quotes (yes he sends me motivational quotes almost everyday). You literally changed your lifestyle by trying to stop bad habits, try to eat healthy, well done. Give yourself a big hand of applause.

It's pretty easy to lose your weight but it's hard for you to lose weight by maintaining muscle growth and fat loss. Right now you are not a beginner anymore as what you thought you are. Just sometimes due to over react or muscle tension gives you stiffness and make the movement slightly off track. But for me overall I can give you 7/10 + 1 (for your effort joining classes on your own will) means you get 8/10 from me.

Please never give up and always chase self development for a better future. Remember ROME was not built in a day so keep up the good habits.

You will undergo a small fitness test before we go for muscle toning. Remember Phase 3 (Maintenance Phase) is not easy because most people fail at this phase. This is why you see people come and go. Challenging Phase.

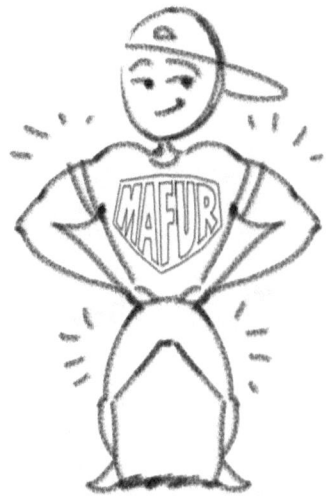

Mr. Mafur... aka Mr. Trainer... aka Muscle Man....

The Author

Jules is a seasoned advertising professional by day (and sometimes night!) and a devoted mom, a kaki makan, and a fitness enthusiast all day long. She started on her fitness journey without even owning a pair of gym shoes, but now she lifts weights, does HIIT, and jumps along with others in workout classes - and feels the best she's ever felt in a long time. Jules is equal parts determined, strong, fierce, and funny; and lives by the mantra "I am woman, hear me roar". She wants to inspire anyone at any age or fitness level to transform their lives because "if she can do it, seriously lah - so can you". This is Jules' first book.

www.ingramcontent.com/pod-product-compliance
Lightning Source LLC
Chambersburg PA
CBHW050422290526
45786CB00003B/1371